RETT SYNDROME
(Genetic disorder)

Rett Syndrome warriors awareness tips

EMILY SMITH

Table of content

Chapter 1:WHAT IS RETT SYNDROME?

(This Rett Syndrome awareness book is completely an information about the infection. It doesn't give clinical exhortation, determination or treatment. This content isn't expected to fill in for proficient clinical exhortation, determination, or treatment. Continuously look for the exhortation of your doctor or other qualified wellbeing supplier with any inquiries you might have in regards to an ailment. Never dismiss proficient clinical exhortation or postpone in looking for it as a result of something you have perused on this book)

Rett Syndrome(genetic disorder):

Rett Syndrome is an interesting hereditary neurological and formative problem that influences the manner in which the cerebrum creates. This problem causes an ever-evolving

alternate ways. They might become impartial in others, toys and their environmental factors. A few kids have quick changes, like an unexpected loss of language. Over the long haul, kids may bit by bit recover eye to eye connection and foster nonverbal relational abilities.

Uncommon hand developments: Kids with Rett condition as a rule foster monotonous, purposeless hand developments, which vary from one youngster to another. Hand developments might incorporate hand-wringing, pressing, applauding, tapping or scouring.

Strange eye developments: Youngsters with Rett disorder will more often than not have surprising eye developments, like extraordinary gazing, flickering, crossed eyes or shutting each eye in turn.

Breathing issues: These incorporate breath holding, fast breathing (hyperventilation), strongly smothering air or spit, and gulping air. These issues will quite often happen during waking hours. Other breathing unsettling influences like shallow breathing or brief times of halting breathing (apnea) can happen during rest.

Peevishness and crying: Kids with Rett condition might turn out to be progressively disturbed and crabby as they age. Times of crying or shouting might start abruptly, for reasons unknown, and keep going for a really long time. A few youngsters might encounter fears and nervousness.

Other strange ways of behaving. These may incorporate, for instance, abrupt, odd looks and long episodes of chuckling, hand licking, and getting a handle on of hair or dress.

Scholarly inabilities: Loss of abilities might be associated with losing the capacity to think, comprehend and learn.

. A great many people who have Rett condition experience seizures sooner or later during their lives. Various seizure types might happen and are related with changes on an electroencephalogram (EEG).

Sideways arch of the spine (scoliosis). Scoliosis is normal with Rett disorder. It normally starts somewhere in the range of 8 and 11 years old and advances with age. Medical procedure might be required assuming the curve is extreme. Unpredictable heartbeat.

This is a dangerous issue for some kids and grown-ups with Rett condition and can bring about unexpected passing.

Issues with rest examples can incorporate unpredictable rest times, nodding off during the day and being conscious around evening time, or waking in the night with crying or shouting.

Different side effects can happen, for example, a diminished reaction to torment; little hands and feet that are normally chilly; issues with biting and gulping; issues with gut capability; and teeth crushing.

Chapter 2: PHASES OF RETT SYNDROME

Rett condition is ordinarily partitioned into four phases:

Stage 1: Early beginning. Signs and side effects are unpretentious and not entirely obvious during the principal stage, what begins somewhere in the range of 6 and year and a half old enough. Stage 1 can keep going for a couple of months or a year. Children in this stage might show less eye to eye connection and begin to lose interest in toys. They may likewise have postpones in sitting or slithering.

Stage 2: Rapid disintegration. Beginning somewhere in the range of 1 and 4 years old, youngsters lose the capacity to perform abilities they recently had. This misfortune can be quick or more progressive, happening over weeks or months. Side effects of Rett condition happen, like eased back head development, unusual hand developments, hyperventilating, shouting or sobbing for reasons unknown, issues with development and coordination, and a deficiency of social collaboration and correspondence.

Stage 3: Plateau. The third stage for the most part starts between the ages of 2 and 10 years, and it can keep going for a long time. In spite of the fact that issues with development proceed, conduct may marginally improve, with less crying and peevishness, and there might be some improvement close by use and correspondence. Seizures might start in this stage and for the most part don't happen before the age of 2.

Stage 4: Late engine disintegration. This stage for the most part starts after the age of 10 and can keep going for years or many years. It's undeniable by diminished versatility, muscle shortcoming, joint contractures and scoliosis. Understanding, correspondence and hand abilities for the most part stay stable or improve marginally, and seizures might happen on rare occasions.

When to see a specialist

Signs and side effects of Rett condition can be unpretentious in the beginning phases. See your kid's medical services supplier immediately in the event that you start to see actual issues or changes in conduct after what gives off an impression of being run of the mill improvement.

Eased back development of your youngster's head or different pieces of the body
Diminished coordination or portability
Monotonous hand developments
Diminishing eye to eye connection or loss of interest in regular play
Postponed language improvement or loss of past language capacities
Any unmistakable loss of recently acquired achievements or abilities

Chapter3:Effects of Rett syndrome

Rett condition is an interesting hereditary problem. Exemplary Rett condition, as well as a few variations (abnormal Rett disorder) with milder or more-serious side effects, happen in light of a few explicit hereditary changes (transformations).

The hereditary changes that cause Rett condition happen haphazardly, for the most part in the MECP2 quality. Not very many instances of this hereditary problem are acquired. The hereditary changes seem to bring about issues with the protein creation basic for mental health. Be that as it may, the specific reason isn't completely perceived and is as yet being contemplated.

Since guys have an alternate chromosome blend from females, guys who have the hereditary changes that cause Rett condition are impacted in obliterating ways. The vast majority of them kick the bucket before birth or in early earliest stages.

A tiny number of guys have an alternate hereditary change that outcomes in a less disastrous type of Rett condition. Like females with Rett condition, these guys are probably going to live to adulthood, however they're currently in danger of various scholarly and formative issues.

Rett condition is interesting. The hereditary changes known to cause the infection are irregular, and no gamble factors have been distinguished. In a tiny number of cases, acquired factors — for example, having close relatives with Rett condition — may assume a part.

Inconveniences of Rett condition include:

Rest issues that make critical rest interruption the individual with Rett condition and relatives.

Trouble eating, prompting unfortunate nourishment and postponed development.

Entrail and bladder issues, like obstruction, gastroesophageal reflux infection (GERD), inside or urinary incontinence, and gallbladder sickness.

Torment that might go with issues like gastrointestinal issues or bone cracks.

Muscle, bone and joint issues.

Nervousness and issue conduct that might frustrate social working.

Requiring long lasting consideration and help with exercises of day to day living.

Abbreviated life length.

Albeit a great many people with Rett condition live into adulthood, they may not live as long as the normal individual as a result of heart issues and other unexpected problems.

Counteraction

There's no known method for forestalling Rett condition. Generally speaking, the hereditary changes that cause the problem happen precipitously.

All things being equal, in the event that you have a kid or other relative with Rett condition, you might need to get some information about hereditary testing and hereditary directing.

Chapter 4:Diagnosis Of Rett Syndrome

Diagnosing Rett condition includes cautious perception of your youngster's development and advancement and responding to inquiries concerning clinical and family ancestry. The determination is generally thought about while easing back of head development is seen or loss of abilities or formative achievements happens.

Rules for determination of abnormal Rett condition might fluctuate somewhat, however the side effects are something very similar, with differing levels of seriousness.

Hereditary testing
In the event that your youngster's medical services supplier suspects Rett condition after assessment, hereditary testing (DNA examination) might be expected to affirm the determination. The test requires drawing a

limited quantity of blood from a vein in your youngster's arm. The blood is then shipped off a lab, where the DNA is inspected for pieces of information about the reason and seriousness of the problem. Testing for changes in the MEPC2 quality affirms the determination. Hereditary directing can assist you with understanding quality changes

In spite of the fact that there is no solution for Rett condition, medicines address side effects and offer help. These may work on the potential for development, correspondence and social cooperation. The requirement for treatment and backing doesn't end as youngsters become more established — it's typically fundamental over the course of life. Treating Rett condition requires a group approach.

Ideal treatment of Rett condition incorporates a multidisciplinary approach that tends to side effects and signs.

A program of word related treatment, exercise based recuperation, and correspondence treatment (with a discourse and language specialist) ought to be given to address self improvement abilities like taking care of and dressing, restricted versatility, strolling trouble, and correspondence deficiencies.

Medications might be expected to control seizures, for breathing brokenness, or for engine challenges.

Customary re-assessment is required for scoliosis movement and to screen cardiovascular irregularities.

Nourishment backing might be expected to assist impacted youngsters with keeping up with weight.

Medicines that can assist youngsters and grown-ups with Rett condition include:

Customary clinical consideration. The executives of side effects and medical conditions might require a multispecialty group. Customary observing of actual changes like scoliosis, gastrointestinal (GI) issues and heart issues is required.

Prescriptions. However prescriptions can't fix Rett condition, they might assist with controlling a few signs and side effects that are essential for the problem. Prescriptions might assist with seizures, muscle solidness, or issues with breathing, rest, the GI parcel or the heart.

Exercise based recuperation. Exercise based recuperation and the utilization of supports or projects can assist youngsters who with having scoliosis or require hand or joint help. At times, exercise based recuperation can likewise assist with keeping up with development, make a legitimate sitting position, and further develop strolling abilities, equilibrium and adaptability. Assistive gadgets, for example, a walker or wheelchair might be useful.

Word related treatment. Word related treatment might work on intentional utilization of the hands for exercises like dressing and taking care of. On the off chance that monotonous arm and hand developments are an issue, supports that confine elbow or wrist movement might be useful.

Discourse language treatment. Discourse language treatment can assist with working on a youngster's life by showing nonverbal approaches to conveying and assisting with social collaboration.

Nourishing help. Appropriate nourishment is critical for sound development and for worked on mental, physical and social capacities. An unhealthy, even eating regimen might be suggested. Taking care of methodologies to forestall stifling or regurgitating are significant. A few youngsters and grown-ups may should be taken care of through a cylinder put straightforwardly into the stomach (gastrostomy).

Conduct intercession. Pursuing and growing great rest routines might be useful for rest unsettling influences. Treatments might assist with further developing issue ways of behaving. Support administrations. Early intercession projects and school, social and occupation preparing administrations might assist with reconciliation into school, work and social exercises. Extraordinary transformations might make cooperation conceivable.

Elective medication

A couple of instances of corresponding treatments that have been attempted in youngsters with Rett condition include:

Music treatment

Knead treatment

Hydrotherapy, which includes swimming or moving in water

Creature helped treatment, for example, restorative horseback riding

Adjusted sports and sporting exercises

In spite of the fact that there's moderately little proof that these methodologies are compelling, they might offer open doors for expanded development and social and sporting improvement.

In the event that you figure option or corresponding treatments could assist your kid, converse with your wellbeing with caring supplier or specialist. Talk about the potential advantages and dangers and how the methodology could squeeze into the clinical treatment plan.

Adapting and support
Youngsters and grown-ups with Rett condition need assistance with most day to day undertakings, like eating, strolling and utilizing the restroom. This consistent consideration and upset rest can be debilitating and distressing for families and can influence the wellbeing and prosperity of relatives.

Track down ways of alleviating pressure. It's normal to feel overpowered now and again. Discuss your concerns with a confided in companion or relative to assist with easing your pressure. Carve out some margin for yourself and accomplish something that you appreciate so you can unwind.

Sort out for outside help. In the event that you care for your kid at home, look for the assistance of outside parental figures who can offer you a reprieve every once in a while. Or on the other hand you might think about private consideration sooner or later, particularly when your kid turns into a grown-up.

Here is a data to assist you with preparing for your kid's arrangement. On the off chance that conceivable, carry a relative or companion with you. A believed sidekick can assist you with recollecting data and offer close to home help.

Any surprising way of behaving or different signs. Your medical services supplier will analyze your youngster cautiously and check for eased back development and improvement, however your day to day perceptions are vital.

Any prescriptions that your youngster takes. Incorporate any nutrients, enhancements, spices and nonprescription prescriptions, and their measurements.

Inquiries to pose to your youngster's medical services supplier. Make certain to pose inquiries when you don't figure out something.

Inquiries to pose could include:

For what reason do you figure my kid does (or doesn't) have Rett condition?

Is there a method for affirming the determination?

What are other potential reasons for my youngster's side effects?

In the event that my youngster really does have Rett condition, is there a method for telling how serious it is?

What changes might I at any point hope to find in my youngster over the long run?

Could I at any point deal with my youngster at home, or will I really want to search for outside mind or extra in-home help?

What sort of extraordinary treatments do youngsters with Rett condition need?

How much and what sorts of customary clinical consideration will my youngster need?

What sort of help is accessible to groups of youngsters with Rett condition?

How might I get more familiar with this problem?

What are my possibilities having different youngsters with Rett condition?

What's in store from your primary care physician

Your medical services supplier might ask you inquiries, for example,

When did you first notification your kid's surprising way of behaving or different signs that something might be off-base?

What might your youngster at some point do before that your kid can never again do?

How extreme are your youngster's signs and side effects? Is it safe to say that they are deteriorating?

What, all things considered, appears to work on your youngster's side effects?

What, all things considered, seems to deteriorate your youngster's side effects?

Your medical services supplier will pose extra inquiries in light of your reactions and your youngster's side effects and needs. Getting ready and expecting questions will assist you with taking full advantage of your arrangement time.

Chapter 5:RETT SYNDROME IN MALES

Guys with Rett-causing transformations for the most part have prior beginning and more serious side effects than females, as every one of the cells in the male have the changed quality. These patients frequently have extreme breathing issues, taking care of challenges, and seizures. They might make due to late adolescence with forceful clinical intercession.

Rett condition was perceived exclusively in females. It was conjectured that Rett condition was deadly in guys. This recommended that Rett condition was a sex-connected hereditary confusion with the quality being restricted on the X chromosome.

In 1999 it was accounted for that transformations in the MECP2 quality, situated on the X chromosome, were related with the clinical show of Rett condition. Since the capacity to test the MECP2 quality has been accessible, there have been more than 60 guys announced with transformations in the MECP2 quality. A couple of these guys had a clinical picture predictable with the clinical standards for Rett condition; be that as it may, the vast majority of these guys gave an alternate clinical show. Most guys with transformations in MECP2 quality present with a previous beginning of side effects, regularly with critical issues starting at or not long after birth.

The determination of Rett condition is as yet in light of clinical standards and the clinical show. More than 95% of females with exemplary Rett condition will have a transformation in the MECP2 quality. Transformations in the MECP2 quality without help from anyone else are not adequate to make a determination of Rett condition. Patients with transformations in the MECP2 quality that don't meet the clinical standards for Rett condition are given the assignment of MECP2-related messes.

The condition is for the most part brought about by transformations in the MECP2 quality situated on the X chromosome and whose capability incorporates controlling the movement of numerous different qualities. Since guys have just a single X chromosome, this implies that a transformation in the MECP2 quality can't be remunerated by a sound quality duplicate. Along these lines, they don't for the most part endure earliest stages.

There are, be that as it may, announced instances of guys with MECP2 transformations. These patients have more extreme side effects that foster right off the bat throughout everyday life, with the principal indications of the infection seen upon entering the world or presently.

In guys, most changes in the MECP2 are because of unconstrained transformations that happen during the division and development of sperm, the male microorganism cell. As the determination of Rett condition depends on clinical standards and show, transformations in the MECP2 quality are not adequate to make a conclusion of Rett. Individuals with such transformations who don't meet the clinical standards for Rett are given the assignment of MECP2-related messes.

There are a few conditions that make sense of the event of Rett disorder in guys. They are:

Klinefelter condition

Klinefelter disorder is a hereditary condition where guys have two X chromosomes notwithstanding their Y chromosome. This condition influences around 1 of every 500 to 1,000 guys.

There is a little opportunity that a kid with Klinefelter condition might have a transformation in the MECP2 quality in one of his X chromosomes that prompts a clinical show predictable with Rett. Notwithstanding Rett side effects, impacted guys additionally have side effects of Klinefelter condition, like immature genitalia and low creation of sex chemicals.

Mosaicism

Mosaicism portrays the presence of two distinct populaces of cells in the body. Each individual begins from one cell, a prepared egg cell. Since each phone in the body emerged from similar unique cell, all phones are hereditarily indistinguishable. This is valid except if a hereditary change or a transformation happens during improvement.

In guys with Rett condition and mosaicism, a few cells have a transformed MECP2 quality while different cells convey a sound duplicate.

The clinical show, and whether side effects are like those found in females, rely upon the level of impacted cells.

MECP2-related serious neonatal encephalopathy Some MECP2 transformations can cause neonatal encephalopathy, a condition described by cerebrum brokenness during earliest stages.

Guys with Rett-causing transformations for the most part have prior beginning and more extreme side effects than females, as every one of the cells in the male have the changed quality. These patients frequently have serious breathing issues, taking care of challenges, and seizures. They might make due to late adolescence with forceful clinical intercession.

Less extreme MECP2 transformations
Some MECP2 transformations don't fundamentally influence the capability of the MeCP2 protein, for which this quality codes. Females with one such transformation for the most part have no side effects or, truth be told, exceptionally gentle ones. In guys, these transformations might cause learning challenges or conduct issues, however not the run of the mill side effects of Rett condition.

Forestalling undernutrition and keeping a solid weight record are significant, as these have been related with better functioning.Surveillance for scoliosis turns into a significant preventive measure; a few youngsters (~20%) eventually require spinal medical procedure for this comorbidity. Longitudinal evaluation of pubertal improvement demonstrates an expanded pervasiveness of early thelarche and adrenarche however postponed menarche. Difficulties with strange tone in this age range ordinarily are described by hypotonia developing to rigidity.

Reconnaissance for scoliosis keeps on being a significant preventive measure, albeit this diminishes with consummation of puberty.Surveillance for urinary maintenance is important.Biliary parcel sickness is found in youthful adulthood at rates like everybody, except because of correspondence debilitation in RTT the introducing side effects might be restricted to peevishness, weight reduction and vomitingStudies of life span in RTT exhibit endurance of numerous into middle age, highlighting the requirement for the early improvement of a far reaching, smart arrangement for progressing to adulthood.Longitudinal management is expected in RTT as physical, conduct and mental impediments won't consider free living.This might incorporate day projects and reprieve care.

Generally speaking, people with RTT will more often than not balance out clinically in youthful adulthood. Frequent reasons for hospitalization for ladies with RTT incorporate pneumonia, respiratory trouble, status epilepticus, rectal dying, decrease in ambulation or refusal/powerlessness to eat or drink.

While 33% of people might have a gastrostomy tube, a big part of these keep on having some oral intake. With age, worry for low bone mineral mass combined with long haul utilization of specific anticonvulsants raises the dangers for osteoporosis and bone fractures,requiring proceeded with supplementation and observing of vitamin D status.

Musculoskeletal issues and gross engine capability might deteriorate overall,potentially because of more parkinsonian features, however safeguarding of keenness and memory, extra review is required because of moderately low numbers contemplated.

Actual restrictions, parkinsonian elements and high pervasiveness of social withdrawal ways of behaving lead to strange or diminished social collaborations predictable with nervousness or depression.

Although most of ladies with RTT in the USA inhabit home, in different nations something like 33% of ladies over age 16 with RTT inhabit home (either full time or parttime), with the greater part residing in a private facility.Long-term and exclusively custom fitted consideration that gives social communications and active work ought to be given at all ages to decrease age-related deterioration.

Chapter 6: The relationship Between Rett Syndrome (MECP2) problems to Autism

Rett Syndrome is a neurodevelopmental disorder (NDD) that is delegated a chemical imbalance range jumble of Autism Spectrum Disorder in the Diagnostic and Statistical Manual of Mental Disorders.RTT is for the most part tracked down in young ladies, albeit few young men have been related to RTT. Albeit mentally unbalanced highlights are available in certain individuals with RTT, particularly during the backward stage, numerous one of a kind clinical elements separate RTT from idiopathic chemical imbalance.

Wide interest in RTT exists in light of the fact that, in 1999, RTT turned into the principal ASD with a characterized hereditary cause. Although most of individuals with RTT have transformations in the X-connected transcriptional controller Methyl-CpG-restricting Protein (MECP2),up to 5% of individuals with RTT don't have changes in MECP2. Now and again, individuals with RTT or RTT-like highlights have transformations in different qualities. Moreover, transformations in MECP2 have been distinguished in individuals who don't have the unmistakable clinical highlights of RTT, yet rather have other brain formative problems (NDDs).

For this explanation, RTT stays a clinical determination characterized by an agreement of clinical criteria. Notwithstanding the deficiency of capability changes in MECP2 that cause RTT, duplication of MECP2 causes a particular NDD,demonstrating that the sensory system is exceptionally delicate to MECP2 portion, and any disturbance in the capability of the protein item, MeCP2, can prompt neurological and mental issues.

The distinguishing proof of the hereditary reason for most of instances of RTT has prompted the improvement of various mouse models of the disease.These models have given significant understanding into the pathophysiology of the problem and point towards conceivable restorative intercessions. Significantly, the creature model has exhibited that the infection is reversible, giving desire to the improvement of treatments that will enhance or totally salvage the sickness.

The numerous clinical highlights found in RTT and the different clinical issues that emerge from disturbing MeCP2 capability has lead the idea that RTT is a "prototypical NDD, that can go about as a Rosetta stone to give understanding and knowledge into an immense range of hereditarily characterized and hereditarily unclear clinical circumstances, for example, idiopathic autism.

To give general data about RTT and MECP2-related messes, this survey will portray the clinical elements of these problems, with an emphasis on the mentally unbalanced highlights present and the one of a kind clinical highlights that characterize these problems. At long last, a concise outline of the creature models of these sicknesses will be introduced and will show how work with these models has prompted the conceptualization and commencement of clinical preliminaries in RTT.

Mentally unbalanced highlights and other conduct issues Autistic elements, for example, social withdrawal and evasion of eye stare happens in certain individuals with RTT, frequently during the time of dynamic relapse (Stage 2).as a matter of fact, an enormous extent of individuals with RTT meet DSM-TV standards for unavoidable formative problem not in any case determined (FDD - NOS), and certain individuals in the long run determined to have RTT are at first determined to have autism.

Leonard and partners observed that the underlying determination of chemical imbalance is more probable in less seriously impacted individuals.

This is predictable with the acknowledgment that medically introverted highlights are more normal in a milder abnormal variation of RTT, the safeguarded discourse variation (PSV).

As a general rule, the medically introverted highlights present during the relapse phase of RTT appear to improve during Stage 3 with expanded and, surprisingly, extraordinary eye stare and interest in friendly communications. In any case, different examinations have found unmistakable highlights of chemical imbalance in RTT that might persevere after regression.

In the main review that deliberately applied an action well defined for mentally unbalanced elements, Mount and partners found that individuals with RTT showed expanded medically introverted highlights contrasted and people with serious scholarly disability.

Utilizing the Autism Behavior Checklist
Using more extensive conduct screening measures, Wulfaett and associates observed that

medically introverted highlights are available in roughly half of individuals with RTT, however these highlights decline with time so 19% at this point not met standards for an ASD.

Recent work utilizing PC based eye-GPS beacons demonstrates that individuals with RTT have an inclination to see human countenances, particularly eyes, which is as opposed to look inclination in autism.

Thus, the specific idea of medically introverted highlights in RTT and their shift over the direction of the sickness stays a critical exploration question that should be efficiently evaluated utilizing suitable measures.
Notwithstanding the mentally unbalanced highlights referenced over, various conduct irregularities have been seen in RTT. One of the most unmistakable is nervousness, which frequently presents as unfortunate articulation and expanded breathing irregularities and hand stereotypies when in a novel and invigorating environment.

Additionally, certain individuals with RTT have self-damaging ways of behaving, for example, head banging, biting on all fours, and hitting themselves.46,48 It has been noticed that individuals with RTT have expanded torment tolerance.

Sometimes individuals with RTT will have explosions of unexplained shouting or laughing.

Finally, rest is extraordinarily disturbed in RTT, with expanded occurrence of trouble nodding off, continuous late-night/early morning feelings of excitement, and expanded daytime napping.

A new report utilizing polysomnography contrasted RTT subjects and controls and found that RTT subjects had expanded quantities of enlightenments each hour of rest and invested a bigger level of energy conscious in the wake of falling asleep.51

In summary

Rett syndrome is an infection with various fascinating clinical highlights, a significant number of which cross-over with other neurological, neurodevelopmental, and neuropsychiatrie messes.

Furthermore, modifications in the capability of the protein result of the quality transformed in many instances of RTT, MECP2, can cause neurodevelopmental messes unmistakable from RTT, including numerous that have mentally unbalanced highlights.

Joined with the accessibility of magnificent creature models this makes RTT and MECP2-related messes not just an interesting and manageable subject for study, however the comprehension that comes from such investigations will probably give understanding into a wide range of neurodevelopmental, neurological, and mental infections.

The commitment given by the reversibility of sickness in the mouse model of RTT has become motivation for the whole neurodevelopmental field and extraordinary expectation exists that restorative choices produced for RTT will demonstrate valuable for other neurodevelopmental messes.